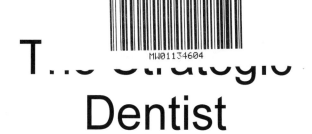

The Strategic Dentist

Dentist

An Entrepreneur's Guide to Starting a Successful Dental Practice

Ali Oromchian, J.D., LL.M.

Here's What's Inside…

DISCLAIMER

The information contained in this book and all related resources are for informational purposes only as a service to the public, and is not legal advice or a substitute for legal counsel, nor does it constitute advertising or a solicitation.

To my mom, Goly, for her devotion
and pure love that knows no bound.

To my wife, college sweetheart, and truest
friend, Ozzie, for her uncompromising
support, encouragement, and love.

To Caroline, Emme and Lily for
you are my life.

Introduction

It is well documented that dental schools typically do not spend much time training their students in business or legal topics. And this absence of business training makes sense as these institutions focus on the clinical practice of dentistry because there is an enormous amount of clinical education that must be transferred in 3 or 4 short years.

After graduation, dentists have access to many resources to further their skills in clinical dentistry but, unfortunately, that has not historically been the case when it comes to the business of dentistry and the steps required to transition from an associate to practice owner.

My goal when I sat down to write this book was to provide a young dentist with a single resource for when he or she is ready to take one of the most important steps of their career: becoming an entrepreneur by either starting or buying a dental practice.

We summarized the most important information that a young dentist needs to know as he or she prepares for practice ownership. Our focus, of course, will be upon teaching you those business-related components of dentistry, which they do not teach you in dental school.

While we won't be able to deep-dive into great detail, our goal is to provide you with enough information so that you can enter into a conversation about practice ownership with a fair amount of knowledge.

We have tried to keep this book very concise, filled with only the most important information that a young dentist asks as he or she begins this process.

We will not turn you into a dental lawyer like me, but rather to give them the meaty information that will allow them to have important conversations with landlords, sellers, and other advisors in a way that is both knowledgeable and strategic. I also address some of the most frequently asked questions that come up during our meetings with our clients.

If you are nervous about opening your own practice or about purchasing one, my hope is that this book will give you the courage to jump into practice ownership feeling equipped with all the information that you need to be successful.

I also hope that by reading this book and using the tools and resources referenced, the guesswork will be taken out of owning a practice so you can build an incredible career helping others, knowing that you are building your practice with a strong legal and business foundation.

To get the most out of this publication, I encourage you to review the checklists we have provided at the end of the book and to reference even more materials at the Strategic Dentist website at http://www.strategicdentist.com including contact information for dental specific consultants, attorneys, CPAs, brokers, financial planners and insurance professionals that you can trust and rely upon.

To Your Success!

Ali Oromchian

My "Why"

If you haven't seen the TED TALK video by Simon Sinek on the power of "Why" I strongly recommend that you search for it on YouTube.

In fact, I urge you to put the book down, go and watch the video and then come back to this section.

…

…

…

I hope you enjoyed the video. So what is my "why"?

I have spent considerable time thinking about this question, as it is not a simple one to answer. But I kept thinking about how helpless we felt when a CPA told my wife that she was committing financial suicide for wanting to become a practice owner so I want to thank him for inspiring me to write this book and I'm proud to say that my why is:

I believe that dentists deserve to play on an even playing field in business and to have the opportunity to become financially independent as they dedicate their life to serve patients. We accomplish this by providing strategic and timely legal advice and counseling in contract and lease negotiations, employment law and business planning.

What Dentists Need to Know in Order to Create a Thriving Dental Practice

While there is no single formula for success in the dental field (or in *any* professional field, for that matter), in order to be a strong entrepreneur and owner of a practice, the dentist will typically need at least two to five years of experience working for someone else after graduation. If they work in a practice that is similar to their ideal practice, then that would be most helpful because they can see how that practice matches some of the initial skills of the practice management side: employee issues, marketing, new patient procedures, referrals, etc.

Obviously, the business needs to be financially healthy as well, which includes excellent credit and other factors reviewed by banks. (Otherwise, the dentist will have been exposed to an *unsuccessful* practice environment and may be poised to start his or her own practice with unhealthy professional habits.)

But owning your own practice has benefits beyond the financial advantages. Owning your own practice means having a say in crucial decisions as to the future of the business. If you have dreamed of "handling things differently," or taking a more modern approach to your practice, owning your own practice is the key to making those dreams a reality. And honestly, readying yourself for incorporating your ideas into your own practice is one of the first steps towards incorporating what we call an "owner mindset" into your day to day role.

Knowing that you possess an owner mindset is key when it comes to owning your own practice, because owners and entrepreneurs must be prepared for the responsibilities that come with being their own bosses. For example, dentists with an owner mindset are not intimidated by the risks and all of the (sometimes unpleasant) issues that accompany ownership. This would include the fact that being an owner of a practice potentially limits your ability to move around with your family and may at first require extended work hours as you find your footing as a new owner. Those with a business mindset understand that they are giving up some of their personal life in exchange for being able to enjoy everything associated with ownership down the road.

OK, so let's get down to the nitty gritty of how you make ownership happen: Basically, there are three options or career choices that will allow you to start building ownership equity. You can either start a practice, buy a practice, or a variation of those two choices such as joining a group practice. You can establish something called a solo group, or you can share space with another dentist. We placed all of those options into one category simply because of the way those things transpire.

Option One - Start a Practice

For many young dentists who dream of practice ownership, starting their own practice is the way that they envision the ownership process taking shape. But building and opening a practice from scratch is not for the faint of heart as it requires a lot of patience, organization and discipline.

Typically, a dental practice of 1,500 to 2,000 square feet can cost anywhere between $350,000 to $500,000 for the tenant improvements, equipment and technology. The process can take anywhere between 6-9 months to complete and may require you to cut down on your associateship which can result in reduced income due to a reduced number of work hours - a caveat that many young dentists do not consider. For example, as an associate, you might be working four days a week (and earning money for those work hours, of course). But becoming a practice owner means that you will starting from the ground up, which requires a significant time investment all on its own. Therefore, you may only be able to work two or three days and be forced to spend the other days focusing on the "busy work" that comes with building your practice.

Also, for most young dentists there is financial pressure created by student loans. Student loans at dentist schools are at the highest level that they have ever been. Because the burden of student loans can make it very difficult for a young dentist to get through even a short period of time without income, some shy away from starting a practice from scratch.

The primary advantage of starting a practice from scratch is that you have choices. You choose exactly where you want to be; and you choose and personalize everything down to the exact design of your office, logo, and equipment. Although the income is slower to grow with a new practice, there are a lot of benefits in starting from scratch.

For example, you are able to say that you were solely responsible for your own success and for everything that you have done to build your practice. This knowledge can be very mentally satisfying and is a large part of the reason many practitioners decide to take on the work of building a practice from scratch.

The negatives, or cons, of a start-up include the expense of the building, the potential lack of income, and uncertainty of success. There may be delays as a result of construction and permits. You may not have a lot of income in the initial years even if you are also working somewhere else. In addition, keep in mind that if you choose to start your own practice from scratch, then the buck stops with you. If you fail, then you really won't be able to blame anybody else. You failed because of what you did or didn't do - or, more specifically, for the choices that you made. We are here to help you navigate your way around this process and to help you avoid some of those bad choices. But when you think about the pros and cons of starting your own practice, this mental pressure is an element that you need to prepare yourself for as well.

The good news is that when we talked to some of the largest dental banks, they tell us that their default rates on loans for dental practices are less than one percent. In and of itself, that is reason enough to jump in and start a practice from scratch (although risks still exist) - that figure is a reassurance that most dentists who choose to start their own practices end up being able to keep their business afloat.

There is no escaping the fact that in the United States, there are a lot of dentists. In fact, it is very rare to find a place with only one or two dentists. However, I encourage you not to be worried about competition when opening a new practice but instead to acknowledge the competition and plan for making that competition irrelevant to your practice.

In this book, I will review a process that you should follow for starting your new practice. The steps that I outline here are provided under the assumption that you are not in an immediate rush and are able to take your time in going through this process. If you are looking to start a practice right away, please read the section entitled "How to Prepare to Start a Dental Practice in 30 Days, located at the end of this book. Regardless if the route you choose, you should continue to review the following information, as it is applicable across the board to those looking to start their own practice.

First, we will provide a general overview, outlining some of the requirements that you will need to meet when beginning the process of starting a practice from scratch. Then we will discuss these steps in more detail later in the book. So, if anything that you read now seems overwhelming, don't worry; we will go through everything step by step as we go along.

The very first step towards starting a practice from scratch is to create a business plan. As a professional who is beginning the process of starting a practice, you must have a very strong understanding of your overall business goals, as well as your future practice's financial projections.

The good news is that your business plan does not need to be 50 pages or contain expert data similar to what a technology company would create when seeking venture capital funding. Instead, it should be concise but filled with important information and data.

So, in terms of creating your business plan, it is important that you identify your mission statement by analyzing your goals and the purpose of your dental practice. This is an important part of the process; however, it is an exercise which is often taken for granted by young entrepreneurs, which is a mistake. If your mission statement is missing or simply filled with generalities, it will negatively impact the marketing message to the community and can significantly detract from your ability to reach your goals.

In this very basic business plan, you write out your goals and your objectives, based on the following questions:

- On what date do you want to open?
- Do you want to try to buy or lease some space?
- Do you want to build or buy an existing practice and renovate it?
- How many employees do you expect to hire?

- What are your long-term plans and growth plans as they relate to your new practice?

- Do you think you will want to grow the practice?

- Will you want to expand it to the point where you might need more space?

- In the future, do you plan on bringing in any associates?

- What are your personal financial objectives? Where do you want to be?

Making these decisions will help you determine the amount of resources you will need and the location of your leased space - both of which are important considerations for your business plan.

Remember, this is a business plan, which is an essential element of starting any new practice. And while it may seem as if we are over-stressing its importance here, you have to remember the role of the business plan in your overall goals. This is your dream; it expresses what you want to achieve overall in your career in small, manageable components.

As one example, you should determine your personal financial objectives by asking yourself, "How much do I want to take home?" Obviously, this number can change over time. For a young dentist, $250,000 might be your goal because that is the kind of number you foresee, but right now, you are only making $100,000 or $150,000. In four years you might have achieved $250,000, so now you want to expand to $500,0000. Aim where you think appropriate; there is no right or wrong answer to this.

The second part, which is one of the more important aspects of this plan, is putting together your strategic advisors. A lot of people talk about putting together a team of advisors, but you have worked too hard just to get standard advisors. You need strategic advisors - professionals who have gone through this process a lot and are looking out for your best interests, trying to get you to another level. To do that, you need to start interviewing experts to determine who is strategic and who is not. Anyone can review a contract or file a tax return. Any dental contractor can build a dental practice, but the question is, are they strategic? Will they take you to another level? Our firm is known nationwide as a group who focuses on helping our partners shift upward. In this book, as we discuss each of the steps required for building a new dental practice (or buying into an existing one), we will be suggesting various strategic advisors who can assist you with each step.

Next, you should start looking at an equipment company to help you with office design. A good equipment representative can visit the location with you, offer their ideas, and help you make decisions about whether the place is a good fit. Start talking to them about supplies and technology, as well as your other office needs, because that impacts your business plan and your business.

Next, it's very important to talk to three professionals: a lawyer, a CPA, and an insurance broker. Those are your core team, obviously along with a bank. Although I may be biased, I do say that the place to start is with your lawyer - have him help by introducing you to people who are very successful with his clients. After your lawyer has introduced a few, you can interview them to see if teach is a good fit or not.

These three are not the only professionals that you will need as you go through the purchase process, but they are the professionals who will remain relevant to your practice long after you have completed the purchase process. Another essential player is your real estate broker; whose involvement is crucial if you are looking to start a practice from scratch.

The third step, now that you've started interviewing your team, is a matter of finding the right space where you will be opening your business. As they say: "location, location, location." After you have identified the city that you would like to target we strongly suggest seeking a demographic study of that city and the surrounding areas. Although most demographic studies will not specifically tell you whether you should open up an office or not, it can give you specific information about that areas which will assist you in deciding whether the city you have picked has a good opportunity for growth for your practice.

As discussed above, the importance of a reliable, knowledgeable real estate broker cannot be overstated. There are a lot of good commercial dental brokers who handle tenant representation; they will help you find a location. It's very important to get a specialist for this work. Your cousin or uncle in commercial brokerage may not be the best person for this job because they may not understand your power and plumbing requirements. Honestly, a lot of commercial brokers don't get paid very much for a 2,000 square foot office, but a specific dental broker can be very, very good in negotiations because they have a lot of experience working only with dentists. Specifically, because dentists are considered high quality tenants, a professional dental broker can negotiate the best possible lease terms on your behalf. In addition, your broker can help to introduce you to other professionals relevant to your practice and can save you a lot of the legwork usually associated with starting a new practice.

If you call us, we would be happy to refer you to a number of very good commercial dental brokers around the country, depending on your location. This broker will show you what's available in your area. You can start looking at the importance of location and also at its visibility to commuters and people walking down the street. To a specialist, this is a lot less of a concern because you're a destination.

Keep in mind that once you find a location, people will refer to you. Once a patient visits your office, they know exactly where you are, so you do not need to be on the busiest street in the downtown area. As a general distance, however, visibility and signage do become very important, depending on your location. Placement in a medical building also becomes very important. One group of our clients are all clustered in this one building; there are probably 15 dentists in this one building, with around 12 of them as our clients, and they're all doing over $1,500,000 in revenue and pushing $2,000,000. Obviously, this setup worked well for them. So, don't be fearful about being in a building with other dentists. Success is more about your own marketing plan and less about competition from other tenants.

As you are identifying the location, you should inventory your competition and decide how you plan to differentiate yourself. Note that while I said that competition should not deter you from starting a practice, you also should not ignore it. If you have done your homework with regard to your mission statement, then this part of the business plan should be fairly simple because you should already have determined what was missing from the dentistry field in your chosen areas and formulated some ideas as how to you can improve upon the existing practices.

Ideally, you should also order a demographic analysis. A few folks can help you with it, and the most common one is Scott McDonald & Associates. They do a really good job with site selection. They will analyze demographics and tell you the number of people in your area with their areas of revenue, so it is well worth the investment.

Once you have chosen a practice, the first step towards securing a business lease is to negotiate a letter of intent. And once that LOI has been accepted by both you and the landlord, the landlord will typically prepare a lease for your attorney to review. In this section, we will discuss leases generally. But for more details about various lease terms and definitions, please refer to the section of this book entitled "The Lease."

If you have not yet hired an attorney at the time in which you would like to submit an LOI, it is important that you do so now. At this stage of the process, you need an experienced real estate attorney. Not only will that attorney protect your interests, but an attorney with extensive experience in real estate is likely to save you time and money in the long term. Also note that it is important for you to hire a dental-specific attorney as there are numerous strategic concepts that should be taken into account when negotiating a dental lease, including what should happen upon an untimely death or disability, state and federal regulatory requirements and increases in rent and other expense obligations.

As you are negotiating your lease, this is the right time to select your equipment specialist and architect. Please note that I've excluded a contractor at this stage because you can't pick a contractor until you have complete blueprint plans from a licensed dental architect.

A strong equipment specialist will be one of your biggest assets as you plan to design and equip your dental practice. They will not only be able to give you a preliminary design to ensure that everything you want is included in the location you have identified, but they also can strategize as to how to maximize your available capital to purchase the equipment and technology you need.

We recommend that you interview and select an equipment specialist from any of the distributors as they can give you realistic numbers for tenant improvements and equipment. You'll see this theme a lot - the importance of seeking help from those with the most experience in their respective fields - and this recommendation starts here, at the very earliest stages of the process.

At this stage of the process, your equipment specialist helps you with preliminary drawings of the office, i.e., how to put six chairs in a 1,500 square foot office, or nine chairs inside of 3,000 square feet. They are fantastic about helping, and most equipment specialists will do this as part of their service for you if you dedicate yourself to them and buy your office equipment from them. That is a great place to start.

In addition, an experienced equipment specialist is also able to work with your lender and your broker. This relationship is essential, because the amount that you are able to invest in equipment is often determined by the amount of your loan. A good equipment specialist can help to explain and justify equipment purchase or lease expenses to as to increase the likelihood of your receiving finances for all of the equipment that you wish to have in your office.

You will have to spend a lot of time with the people you hire, working very closely together, because you have to figure out the answers to a lot of questions, such as:

- Where will the receptionist sit?
- What are the size requirements for the rooms?
- Will you offer general anesthesia?
- Do you want to add specialists in the future?
- How many chairs do you want for hygiene?

A good equipment specialist will also talk to you about power. This is always forgotten by people who are not specialists and don't rely on them. You must have at least 200 amps of power for your dental practice - not 100 amps and not 150. Some disastrous situations have been caused when the commercial broker and the contractor have forgotten to check, and every other professional has forgotten to check, so the dentist signed the lease without being able to use all of his equipment. Make sure you have access to your 200 amps of power.

Plumbing is also very important. You need to meet certain plumbing requirements for your county and district for a professional practice. At that point, while negotiating the details of the office lease, you should also be talking to a contractor and an architect; even though the equipment company will be doing the design, the architect and/or the contractor will be involved in the interior design portion and perhaps the traffic flow of the office.

In our experience, architects can be very advantageous to the process, but sometimes getting them on board prolongs the timeframe for getting your location prepared for housing your practice. We usually say that if you hire an architect, add two or more months to your construction time, whereas if you do design-build with a contractor you can reduce the time by two months. That means moving from a four to six-month project to a six to nine-month project as a result, so just keep that in mind.

That being said, hiring an architect can be a wonderful decision for those looking to start a practice from scratch. The architect is responsible for the overall design of your practice. He or she also obtains permits and oversees the work of the engineers, contractors and suppliers. The architect holds everyone accountable to budgets and deadlines, and that your resulting space encompasses your vision for your practice.

After the architect has analyzed your space and come up with a plan (with your approval, of course), the design should be almost completed at that point. If you timed it strategically, then you can begin construction, which is important for the timeline. You're not off the hook since there is still a lot to do during the construction stage and preparing for your opening day, but that's the process for starting your office from scratch.

Finally, the budget and capital requirements for your project should be analyzed, including a cash flow analysis for your personal expenses.

Here are some final questions to ask yourself as you prepare to open your new practice:

1. Have you done a personal and practice budget?

2. Have you performed a demographic study?

3. Have you submitted the paperwork to insurance companies?

4. Have you created a marketing plan?

5. Do you have an on-site project manager for your construction?

Returning to your lease, you will need to create the legal entity that will be the official "tenant" in this document. In other words, you need to determine the legal name (and legal status) for your new business. We always recommend choosing to form a corporation, but sometimes limited liability companies are appropriate. For more details on this complicated step, see the section below entitled **"Legal Entities That Protect You."**

You should finalize the selection of your architect once your lease is fully executed. Depending on how much work you've already done with your equipment specialist, it may take 30-60 days to finalize the blueprints from your architect. This timeline is very important because you should not get bids from contractors until the final plan is ready, including the selection of all fixtures and design elements. Following this process will ensure that you minimize (or, ideally, eliminate) change orders or unexpected increases in your construction costs.

Choosing a contractor becomes much simpler if you have retained the services of an architect. The architect can recommend reliable contractors and keep them on time and within budget without requiring you to micromanage the process. If you decide not to use an architect, then your broker should be able to recommend some reliable contractors as well.

After you have selected your contractor from 2 or 3 bids, the construction will begin. But this does not mean that your job is done. In fact, it is beginning as you must now plan on working on your licenses, permits, and insurance. We have provided a checklist at the end of this book which breaks down in detail some of the licenses, permits and insurances you must have prior to your opening day.

One of the most crucial moments in your practice startup phase is about 1 month before you open your doors. The reason this is a crucial moment is because it is also one of the main times during which young dentists can get in hot water: We're talking about human resource violations. In fact, in my law practice we see more employment law complaints filed against our dentists than malpractice claims – this is true even if you add in cases against oral surgeons who historically have the highest claims of *alleged* malpractice. If you think about it, that is a very surprising bit of information which demonstrates just how dangerous human resource violations really can be.

On average, there are 12-18 documents that you must have completed and signed by every employee once you begin the hiring process. These documents, along with an employment handbook, are the foundation to ensure HR compliance and effective performance management. That is why you need to start thinking about and generating these documents early on.

The reality is that getting an employment handbook and the new hire documents is really just the beginning of the conversation. We have noted a trend between the most successful practices and their use of technology such as CAD/CAM, lasers, Cone Beam 3D and paperless practice management systems, and in the HR context we have identified that successful practices rely on a complete HR solution that not only gets them to compliance but also helps improve employee performance in a paperless environment that is completely integrated with time clocks, benefits tracking, performance reviews and task management. What all of that means, essentially, is that the earlier you begin thinking about your HR needs and correctly implementing a system that is going to work best for you, the better off your practice will be once it opens its doors.

We recommend HR for Health for all startups as their compliance tools and affordable pricing is a "no-brainer" for new practices. In addition, their metrics for employee performance increases productivity to levels that have made HR for Health the go-to software for many consultants, state associations and dental distributors. They succeed because they are experts in their field, and they can help you to make up for any lack of business-related information that you did not receive in dental school.

Also, in this final month prior to opening your doors, it is important that you develop a marketing and community outreach plan. We recommend using a dental consultant to help you craft those strategies as they can help you avoid making mistakes that others have made before you. You'll quickly learn that there truly is no reason to reinvent the wheel when services such as this can be purchased with a measured return on investment.

I hope the above suggestions and others found throughout this book empower you to consider opening a new practice, as it can provide you with the opportunity to open the practice of your dreams. The work will be difficult, but the payoffs can be incredible.

Option Two – Buy a Practice

In addition to starting a practice from scratch, you can also become a practice owner by buying a practice. Buying, or taking over a practice, especially if you're already working at the practice that you are looking to purchase, is really one of the best strategies.

If you already know (or believe) that your supervising dentist is willing to sell to you, then you should seriously consider this route as an option. Unlike buying into some other practice where you have never worked, you have some great advantages that reduce some of the risk associated with new practices: patients know you. Ideally, you've seen the patients for one or two years. The team knows you and they're likely to stay after the transition. As part of the community, you likely know what is and what is not working in terms of that practice's success. All of these advantages explain why buying a practice is generally regarded as being a lower risk strategy than starting a practice from scratch.

Regardless of which route you choose, there will always be aspects to buying practices that you can just never know 100% in advance. That is part of the risk with starting any practice, regardless of whether you're buying in or starting from scratch. However, if you have already worked in the practice, your risks are a lot smaller than when buying a practice where you have never worked. Those practices require more work up-front, such as due diligence on things to watch for and focus on when you are buying someone else's practice, so that you can decide whether that practice is really the right one for you.

We always tell our clients that they will need professional assistance whenever they either start from scratch or buy another person's practice, because all purchase routes have their own advantages and disadvantages. For example, one of the disadvantages in buying an existing practice is that you don't necessarily have the ability to change many things or change them quickly. It might take you a little bit longer to implement changes because the existing team may not appreciate them; you don't want to upset the team and have them leave. Nor do you want the patients concerned that you're changing the practice because they naturally start thinking about whether or not you're charging them more for updating the wallpaper and carpet as well as the equipment with new technology. Certain modifications are considered either acceptable or not acceptable to do, just because of people's perception (both the team and your future patients) and the possibility of going overboard, so it is usually a good idea to just stick to a few changes at a time.

The good news is that when you decide to buy a practice, there are special consultants and commercial brokers in the business of selling practices who can either act for the seller or act for the buyer (as your agent). That's very helpful because you will need assistance.

The big pro of buying in is that there is a very small amount of risk - the practice is already in existence and is likely already successful. The investments and short-term lending, what you are spending at the practice, usually should pay for themselves in very short order because of the way that dental practices are transacted and valued. You will gain some management experience because your team members are already working in the office, and it is a definite positive that you are not working alone in the business. You can get a lot of support from the rest of the team, and hopefully from the seller as well.

The negative aspect of buying a practice is that the buying process can be very slow sometimes, in terms of the legal machine and negotiating the deal. The documents can be hand-picked by the seller because the current market is very seller-friendly. Depending on if you are buying in or buying out someone, you may not be in charge or you might still be the minority owner. Some components of that process can develop which you might later discover to be a disadvantage.

If you have decided not to start a practice from scratch, that you want to buy someone else's practice, the LOI for the lease is slightly different. It's also non-binding, except for confidentiality and other specific items. Signing the LOI does not mean that you have to buy it, but again, the same cautionary tale applies. Don't sign the LOI unless you're absolutely sure that you will buy the practice.

Purchase Structure: These are the questions that must be determined before you move forward.

- Are you buying in as a corporation?
- Are you buying in as an LLC?
- Are you buying stock (not recommended)?
- Are you a partner?

Price of Payments: Terms also need to be stated in the LOI when you're buying a practice. It should cover the way you will handle accounts receivables and excluded assets, but there should be no language about assumptions of liability - you don't want to assume any liabilities from the seller.

Post-Closing Transition Period: How many months or weeks will the seller transition with you? It's very important to be available by phone or in person.

Noncompetition and Nonsolicitation: This is the next item. In almost every state, you can allow a seller to, or you can add a dot-com physician agreement to your contract, in order to prevent a seller from competing against you. This makes sense because you don't want somebody to sell you a business and then go open up a few doors down the street or the shopping center and take back all of the patients.

However, the duration and the area must be reasonable. You cannot say the entire state of Georgia or New York. It has to be a geographically limited area and occurring over a number of years. Usually, the contracts will state between five to 20 miles as the geographic area, and five years as the specific duration.

Confidentiality: This must be present during the negotiations. I always recommend adding a 'no shopping provision' so the seller can't go shopping the idea to other buyers. Sometimes if a broker is involved, they do not like that very much because they take backup offers. However, you can slightly vary the language to say that backup offers can be considered but the seller cannot shop it and exclude the buyer (you) because you have not yet signed the final contract. This does happen, usually when brokers are not involved, because brokers of dental workers are very strong and very good at what they do. They care about buyers just as much as they care about sellers, but sometimes without a broker involved, this happens.

Practice Valuation: This is the next step after the LOI has been completed. Usually, you'll receive a practice valuation by a dental broker or CPA. It's very important to show this valuation to your own CPA to verify the numbers, and make sure that it's within the line or brackets of what's typical in your state. The good news is that it is a discussion of cash flow, so practice valuations fall under definite ranges, but they can increase or decrease depending on the amount of technology and the age or newness of your office. If you have a CAD/CAM, your own cameras, and your paper list, you will be paying more for your practice than if the practice includes paper charts, no computers, and the building is very old.

A quick comment: For a more extensive discussion of how to properly valuate a practice you wish to purchase, please see the section on practice valuation in the next chapter, "Option Three - Joining a Group or Partnership. While buying into a practice and taking over an existing one are two different methods of ownership, they share a number of processes, including valuation and the LOI. Therefore, even if you are certain that you will be taking over a practice as opposed to buying into one, it is still highly recommended that you read the following chapter in order to learn as much as possible about these important steps.

Cash Flow: This really means that your bank and CPA should be doing an analysis of the net amount of money you will have earned at the end of the day after you have paid all of your expenses in the practice, and paid the lender the loan amount owed for purchasing the practice. Then the amount left over is for you. Banks do their cash flow analyses because it's their money they're lending. Your CPA will definitely do an analysis as well.

Truthfully, cash flow numbers sometimes amount to less than what you made as an associate. That can be fine if you give yourself a timeline because it's a strategic decision. "For the next two or three years [whatever it is for that practice], I will make less." In buying a practice, you will often get paid less at the beginning but in you'll be paid more over the long term. If you don't look at it that way, if you get paid less as an owner than you were paid as an associate, that's probably a bad deal for you.

Due Diligence: When buying a practice, it's important to 'do your due diligence,' which basically means your homework on the practice. There are a few things to gather. Financial information is vital, so you have to gather certain documents from the practice: tax returns, profit, and loss balance sheets, practice management software data, etc. The practice management software data should show how many patients made appointments, the types of insurance taken, the age of the patients, etc. All of those things are vital because they need to be verified by you and by your CPA. If a practice is bringing in $1,000,000, with $600,000 earned from placing implants and doing Invisalign®, but you don't like to place implants and you are not an Invisalign® provider, that practice is not right for you even though it is making $1,000,000.

Due diligence options have been extremely important for our clients. Some CPAs will want to verify deposits, so they will review the practice management software about the dentists' earnings and then ask to see a bank account where those deposits get deposited. That's a strong idea if you have the time to do it, and some CPAs definitely do. Check the practice facility, especially if you are going to own the building. We already covered leases.

Operational issues are also part of your due diligence.

- How does this team operate?
- How does it communicate?
- Who's the manager?
- Who are the associates?
- What is the relationship like?

Most of the employee material will not be disclosed to you until you're further down the process, so just be ready for that, because they want to make sure that you'll actually be buying. However, it is okay to ask questions.

Here are some final questions to ask yourself as you prepare to buy a practice:

1. Do you have a marketing plan?
2. Did you review patient charts in your due diligence?
3. Are you satisfied with the financials and has your CPA verified the tax returns and the practice management data?
4. Have you interviewed the employees?
5. Has your attorney reviewed the lease and ensured that you have options to extend?

6. Have you spoken to dental consultants to assist in your due diligence?

Option Three – Joining a Group or Partnership

With the above information about buying into a practice being said, a third option for practice ownership is that you can join a group. They might have an institution already set up with a partnership incentive; maybe only one of those partners is selling, and you could have the option to buy that person's interest. A partnership is also possible if somebody stays with you, such as a mentor, for example. But you should know that partnerships can be difficult when you're joining a team; the relationship is a bit like a marriage. You're getting into a relationship with someone that might last 20 to 30 years, meaning that you've got to really know that person.

There can be buy-in options with a really big group, also called a 'solo group', and this option usually has a different way of dealing with expenses. In a solo group, each member of the group is a solo practice; you have your own practice, and everybody else has their own practice, but you all share expenses. You benefit from sharing expenses, which lowers your overhead. Each owner takes responsibility for his or her own patients. Those solo groups have some advantages as well, but again, you are getting into a partnership in some ways, so you really have to do your homework.

One of my favorite options for younger dentists is something called a 'space-sharing agreement'. Once you find someone who's willing to share their space, you rent from them the opportunity to use some of their chairs, maybe on days when the practice is closed. If the practice is big enough, perhaps a six-chair practice, maybe you could rent their chairs on open days; perhaps you're just using three of the chairs while the other dentist uses three chairs, or you're using two chairs while the other dentist uses four chairs.

Space-sharing is a good way to start slowly and to minimize risk without a great deal of investment, and you can build from there. It is a great way of minimizing risk while you grow your patient pool. You may outgrow the other dentist's space, and then you can start building out a practice or buying someone else's practice while bringing in your own patients. There are many different possibilities and opportunities when you start out in this way.

Unfortunately, it can be very difficult to find people who are willing to share space, very similar to renting and having a roommate live in your house. A lot of dentists spend more time in their offices than in their own home, which means that if they share their office, they now have a roommate at work. You have to let them use the cabinets, use the equipment, and other business tools, so sharing is a big part of your everyday life.

Buying into a practice is completely different from starting one from scratch or buying a practice from someone else. That's because, when you start a new practice or take over an existing one, you will eventually be running a business on your own, in most circumstances. Buying into a practice, however, requires that you become part of a team. Plus, while there is nothing really stopping you from starting your own practice or buying one that is for sale, buying into a practice is a process over which you will have only limited control.

First, you must determine whether the practice is even in the market for another partner. And even if they are, then you need to know whether you are the person that they want to fill that role. Unless the answer to both of those questions is yes, then you will not be buying into the practice, no matter how much you may want to do so.

Most people who buy into a partnership are doing so because they have worked, or are working at that same practice. This strategy makes sense, given that the existing partners already know you and have experience working with you, and because your history with this practice will provide insight into whether seeking a partnership in this practice would be a good decision for you.

Assuming that this is your first time buying into a practice, you may be unsure of where to start. Unless you have been directly approached about becoming a partner, you may have to do a little detective work to see if the practice is interested in adding another partner in the first place. One way to do that is to pay attention to any casual remarks about partnership opportunities from the owners. If you feel comfortable doing so, then you should pull him or her into a private office and "unofficially" ask about the opportunity. This should be a very informal conversation. You are really just looking to determine whether the practice is open to a new partner, and if so then what kind of timeframe they may be looking at as far as making a decision.

If it sounds like the practice is interested in taking on another partner, then that is great news. But remember that just because they want a partner doesn't necessarily mean that that partner will be you. If there are associates who have been with the practice for a longer period of time, for example, then they might have seniority. Even if that is true, however, that doesn't mean that those associates who have seniority are even interested in, or capable of, becoming a partner. Because you *are* interested in seeking a partnership, this is when it becomes important for you to advocate for yourself. Remember that buying into a practice is a two-way street: while you are determining whether you want to buy into partnership, you are also presenting yourself in the best light possible so as to increase the likelihood that they accept your buy-in proposal.

Therefore, if other associates have seniority over you but you are certain that you wish to pursue a partnership - and you are fairly certain that the practice is in the market for a partner, then you should start thinking about ways that you can distinguish yourself from the other associates and show that you are the best choice for the position. One way that you can do this is by drafting a proposal that shows that you are serious about pursuing partnership, and that you are willing to take steps towards making a financial investment into the practice.

Therefore, your first step in demonstrating that you are serious about pursuing partnership is to draft a proposal and begin to seek out financing options.

While we will discuss the specifics of your financing options in more detail below, you should know that financing a partnership buy-in is often different from the financial options used to purchase a practice from someone else or to start one from scratch. That is because when you are buying into a practice, owner financing is often an option. At this stage, however, even if you might prefer an owner-financed deal, coming to the practice with your own financing in place is a very strong option if you are able to pursue that route. Personal savings, family loans, and small business loans are great options for creating a draft proposal. Ultimately, the practice might end up financing the buy-in, but having your own money indicates that you are ready for the responsibility of business ownership. So, if that is something that you are able to bring to the table, mentioning it in your draft proposal is a great way to increase your chances of being chosen for partnership.

Speaking of finances, as part of your draft proposal you will have to discreetly determine a general value for the business. It is recommended that you look into this issue as privately as possible, because If anyone in the practice catches on that you are drafting a partnership proposal, your opportunity could get cut short by office politics - especially if there are more senior associates in your practice. Note that what you are seeking now is not an official valuation which would take place further down the line if your draft proposal is well-received. This valuation is simply used as part of your efforts to demonstrate the sincerity of your buy-in interests is more of a preliminary, generalized valuation used simply for your purposes in drafting your proposal.

By providing some simple information, a professional appraiser can give you a general value for the practice. This evaluation won't be exact, of course, but part of the benefits of drafting the proposal is simply showing the current owners that you know how to put together a business package.

Once you have a reasonable appraisal of the business (or of other like-sized practices, if you are unable to obtain specific figures for your practice) and once you have a general idea of your financing package (personal finances and small-business loan options), you can approach one of the practice owners - preferably the one you know and get along with the best. While you may be anxious to demonstrate your serious interest in partnership, it is recommended that you let your proposal do the talking at this point. Being too aggressive at this stage could hurt your chances.

Keep in mind that the goal is to encourage the current owners to see you as an asset, which they would like to add to their team. Therefore, you should never threaten to leave the practice, or make overt comments about how maybe your skills would be better appreciated someplace else. The reason that you are pursuing partnership is because you enjoy working at this practice. And if that is not the case, then you should not be seeking to buy into this practice in the first place. But assuming that you do enjoy working there, they buying into the practice allows you to keep working with your established staff, to continue seeing your same patients, etc. In other words, it is to your benefit to make this work. So you should do your best to avoid taking any actions, which could jeopardize your chances.

And remember, the current owners know how difficult it is to find someone who wants to buy into a practice. They should want to bring you on as a partner as much as you want to become one. But it is best to allow them to reach this conclusion on their own, rather than aggressively trying to make the point for them.

What if You Change Your Mind About a Buy-In?

As you start the buy-in process, it is normal for you to have some doubts about your decision. Making the change from associate to partner is a big one, and just drafting the proposal and waiting to measure the other owners' interest in your offer can be stressful. So if you are starting to have cold feet, don't panic. Throughout my years of helping dentists become owners, I have yet to have a client who goes on to regret the decision. Still, this is often the point in the process when I start to field questions from clients as to whether they can change their minds once they have started the buy-in process. Therefore, in case you find yourself having these same questions, we will not turn to the issue of whether buying into a practice is, or must be, a permanent decision.

The answer is that buying into a practice is a semi-permanent decision. When you are buying into a practice, you are likely locking yourself into the business for a decade. If you later change your mind, you can get out of the practice in less than ten years. Unfortunately, doing so may require some financial sacrifices. That's because the buy-in purchasing process is *intended* to be permanent due to financing and goodwill considerations. Getting out of a practice in fewer than ten years essentially ensures both monetary and goodwill options.

Here is why. Unless you have a significant amount of cash on hand to buy 20% of the practice outright, you will need to finance the deal. For example, let's say that buying into your practice costs $200,000.00 and that you secure the entirety of that cost with owner financing. Over the course of ten years, that comes to $20,000 per year, or $1,666 per month plus interest. Like with any large loan, you are likely to be paying more of the interest up-front.

When your payments are directed towards the interest, this structure forces you to continue working in the practice until the interest is paid and you actually start to gain equity in the business (by making payments toward the principal). On a ten-year finance buy-in, you might spend three years or more paying back the finance loan before you start to see any real ownership in the practice. If you exit before you gain equity, then you will have been wasting all of those payments. Therefore, the longer you stay, the more equity you gain.

The other issue to consider when you look at leaving a practice after starting your buy-in is the loss of goodwill. Goodwill is a business term which refers to a company's overall value as a brand. For you as a partial owner, the more time you spend working as a partner, the more experience (or goodwill) you have personally. In other words, the longer that you stay with your practice as an owner, the more value that you have to that practice.

Generally speaking, this is how business goodwill works: Once you become a partner, you will be assigned a specific aspect of the business to oversee. For example, let's say that you become responsible for the human resources components of the practice. While there might be an office manager to handle any day-to-day decisions, as the go-to partner for human resource issues, you would be responsible for buying the annual health plan, hiring and firing decisions, and setting up a bonus structure. These responsibilities, of course, are tasks which are not customarily taught in dental school; therefore, you will learn about these tasks while you are working as an owner, and these processes will become easier for you the more time that you spend completing them.

As time passes and you've been working at the practice as an owner for several years, you will have become the expert on human resources issues. In addition, as a partner, you will have a general understanding of other aspects of the business such as marketing, facilities, and medical compliance. If you choose to leave after a few years, the practice loses your expertise. Even if you successfully sell your portion of the practice to a new partner, that person won't have your years of specific experience. This is how your *goodwill*, or value to the practice, increases over time. The earlier you leave your practice, the less time that you will have to build this goodwill and increase your value as a partner.

This concept also applies to your patient base. The longer you stay with your practice, the larger your loyal patient base will be. If you have a group of dedicated patients with whom you have built a relationship and established trust, then the higher the likelihood that those patients would follow you if you chose to leave your practice. In other words, your number of dedicated patients comprise a value which contributes to your overall value as a partner. The earlier you leave, the lower your goodwill in terms of your dedicated patient base.

The bottom line is that no buy-in is truly permanent. And most partnership plans come with an exit strategy designed for retirement, for example. However, given the potential losses that you face were you to choose to leave early, it is in your best interest to stay in your ownership role at a particular practice for as long as possible. You should take this information into account when it comes to formulating a mindset for approaching your buy-in offer. To put it simply: If you are thinking about becoming a partner, make sure you are ready to stay put for at least ten years. Never make a buy-in decision on a whim: it is one that will affect your life for a good amount of time to come.

Buy-In Financing Options

So, assuming that you have decided to move forward with your buy-in proposal, the next issue that must be addressed is financing. Generally, you will have four resources for financing a partnership buy-in: 1. personal finances; 2. business loans; 3. personal loans; and 4. owner financing. While some associates are able to accomplish a buy-in using their own personal finances, most dentists making the transition from associate to partner will use third party financing.

Personal Financing

Personal financing is just what it sounds like: using the funds that you personally have on hand to invest into the business via your buy-in. The amount of your required personal investment varies from practice to practice.

One of the biggest benefits of using your personal finances to cover part of the buy-in price is that it reflects financial responsibility. No one wants a business partner running away from defaulted student loans, credit card write-offs, and a house in foreclosure. If you can't keep your own finances in some semblance of order, no business is going to welcome you as a partner. You will need to survive a credit check, and if you think that you cannot do so, then becoming a partner is not the right decision for you at this time. Instead, you should focus on putting your own debts in order and reconsider partnership when your financial circumstances have improved. Again, the importance of strong financial responsibility is a component of dentistry which would not have been taught in dental school, but which can make or break your goals of becoming a practice owner.

Business Loans

If you find yourself needing to borrow part of your practice buy-in from a commercial lender, then you will likely discover that this is not a difficult process. Dental practices are a reliable business model and you are likely to find several lenders and business loan options for your buy-in. In order to qualify, however, you will need to meet credit standards and will have to have the ability to finance part of your buy-in with personal funds. As you are shopping for a lender, keep in mind that your business loan options might be limited by the pre-approved banks set by the practice owners. Because your lender will have to sign off on the dental practice, you should not necessarily assume that your desired lender would approve the practice.

Also, if you are told to find your own lender, then you should not simply do a Google search in order to research your options. Finding a lender is a great opportunity to visit www.strategicdentists.com and asking for a referral as many lenders provide offers to our readers that is not available to the public. Your future partners are also great referral resources, and you may even be able to get a better rate by using a lender who already has a solid connection to your practice.

Because most dental lenders provide 100% financing to dentists, this is typically the ideal solution.

Personal Loans

Assuming that you need to borrow the majority of the funds needed for your buy-in, there is no requirement that you borrow those funds from a traditional lender or via owner financing. If you have friends or family members who are able to loan you the money, then this is a perfectly acceptable option to use as long as you disclose the source of the loan to your fellow owners as part of the buy-in application process and the owners approve of your lender. Typically, the dental practice will approve this kind of loan as long as the lender (your friend or relative) doesn't receive any kind of ownership in the business if you default on payments. Therefore, in addition to disclosing the source of your loan, you also must disclose your repayment arrangements. And yes, even if you are borrowing the money from friends or family members, you need to establish official repayment arrangements up front. You should consult your attorney for assistance with this process.

Keep in mind that personal loans are sometimes risky because borrowers are more likely to justify a default. Think about it - if you find yourself in a financial bind, you are more likely to make your car or mortgage payment before taking care of repaying a loan to a rich aunt. And especially if your family member is laid back about receiving payments, then this can lead to a risky position, where you get in a habit of failing to repay the loan. And while failing to repay any type of loan is risky, failing to repay a family member or friend can lead to intra-family turmoil. You can avoid those risks by using personal funds, business loans, and/or owner financing in lieu or personal loans.

If you DO accept a personal loan, treat it as you would any other, and honor your repayment obligations.

Owner-Financing

Finally, if personal loans are not an option and you do not have the funds on-hand to cover the full price of the buy in, and you do not wish to use an outside commercial lender, then you will need to use the owner-financing option, in which the practice essentially loans you the funds you need for the buy-in. From the practice's perspective, this option is advantageous for two reasons – high return on investment and control of finances.

The practice itself will make money on your loan via the interest charged. Your fellow owners are more likely to want your interest payments to go toward the practice as opposed to simply being paid to a bank, for example. Plus, because the practice is structuring the loan, the practice can dictate all of the loan terms. For example, the practice can charge a higher interest rate because the loan is guaranteed to be issued, allowing you to avoid the inconvenience of an underwriting process. Owner financing also ensures that the practice can dictate the interest repayment scheme.

The second advantage to the current practice owners is that the practice can take its loan payment each month before issuing you your paycheck, essentially guaranteeing repayment of this loan over the course of your employment. This option is incredibly convenient to you as well, of course. With an internal loan, you might not even notice a change in your paycheck, because internal financing is often designed to create a slight annual bump in pay when an associate becomes a partner. Each year, the new partner makes a bit more money than the last, and at the end of the loan period (generally ten years) the partner is fully vested.

As with any other type of loan, the practice will want to check your credit worthiness and may request a down payment to ensure you remain dedicated to being a partner. Overall, owner financing is a lending option which can be advantageous both to you and to the practice, making it a sound choice for your buy-in payment although there are definitely risks as well.

Practice Valuation:

In order for you to buy a percentage of any dental practice, you and the current owners have to come to an agreement over the current value of the entire business. You can't buy an interest in anything unless you know what the entity is worth. In some cases, the current owners will have a strong grasp the value of the practice. For example, the current owners might routinely borrow money against the value of the business. Borrowing money to invest in the business would mean underwriting evaluations by banks, and the owners would then have an idea of the value based on external evaluation. Similarly, if the owners have recently seen the addition (or withdrawal) of a partner, they will at least have a notion of the evaluation process – if not a solid number to use as a basis for the overall worth.

If you are buying into a smaller dental practice, however – or any-sized practice with less experience in practice valuation – you might have a bit of a battle on your hands in coming to an agreement with the current owners over the value of the business. Generally, a business owner will see his or her business as worth far more than the numbers say. Not only do most business owners rarely take a mile-high view of the finances, but most business owners also have an emotional stake in their business that investors and independent valuators simply don't have.

Inversely, a long-standing business has "goodwill." Goodwill is an accounting term used to cover the financial valuation gap between a business's worth on paper and the value of the business's reputation. As a new partner, you have to concede some additional value to the business because of its long-standing reputation as reliable dental practice. What this means is that the business will actually be "worth" more than simply its on-hand assets. To understand the concept of goodwill, think about the price difference between generic Cola and Coke. If given the opportunity to choose, many consumers would pay $1 for a can of Coke instead of just 75 cents for the generic brand. There's a very good chance the soda is very similar (if not exactly the same), however consumers are often willing to pay more in order to ensure they are going to get exactly what they want. This is due to the *goodwill* that Coke has built with consumers over time.

Before you and your potential business partners set a dollar amount, establish a system by which everyone will agree on the value of the business. You should insist on an external valuation almost without exception. Unless the business has undergone an unbiased evaluation within the last 18 months, there are too many variables that deserve consideration for this process to be managed by anyone other than an outside, disinterested entity.

This evaluation process is also an important opportunity for you to understand the financial underpinning of the business. As a future owner, you will be making decisions based on these very factors and being involved in the evaluation process will mean you will have a stronger, more knowledgeable voice sooner than later.

Due Diligence

Due diligence literally means doing your part to investigate an issue in order to protect yourself. But when it comes to buying into a dental practice, due diligence means you are going to look for any secrets that the company or the partners would prefer remain hidden. This makes for a sensitive subject area. However, uncovering any undisclosed information can mean that you will have a stronger position for negotiating the price of the buy-in. Unfortunately, due diligence could also reveal information that could make you seriously second guess the decision to buy in at all. Still, it is a step that needs to be taken by anyone looking to buy into a dental practice, regardless of the potential risk of uncovering unfavorable information.

In business and finance, due diligence is a common way to feel secure that you are investing your money while being fully informed about where your money is going. Due diligence is also a responsible choice, allowing you to invest your money knowing that it isn't being funneled into a company which is practicing in illegal or otherwise unscrupulous operations.

Financial Due Diligence

Financial due diligence is a form of forensic accounting. Generally, you will have to hire an independent accountant to review the company's most recent financial statements and tax filings. If there is something shady going on with the company's money, you aren't likely to see it in the financials that they present to you as part of the offer. However, a good forensic accountant will be able to detect anomalies and red flags that you can use as a leveraging point in your negotiations.

Dental practices are generally not the kind of business that acts as the front for money laundering operations. So generally, you should ask the forensic accountant to review the tax statements. Dental and medical practices usually don't have to invent significant expenses to write down the taxable profits. However, if gone unchecked for many years, you could be buying into a practice where the partners have become comfortable writing off far too many personal expenses as business costs. Frequently, write offs that start as legitimate expenses can spiral into fraudulent entries when included in the company's business tax returns. As a partner, you will be signing off on those tax returns in the future. You should know ahead of time if you could be facing an uphill battle in order to avoid tax evasion charges.

If the company refuses to hand over any financial statement prior to the buy-in, consider that a significant warning sign. Ultimately, if something illegal is going on inside the company's financial maneuvers, you become a party to it once you are a partner. An official report from a forensic accountant will act as an insurance policy for you in case a problem emerges in the future.

Legal History

Generally, private investigators perform legal due diligence searches. Going back ten or fifteen years, these kinds of reports show any lawsuits in which the dental practice was named as a plaintiff or defendant. A thorough search requires investigating civil and criminal courts at the local (city), municipal (county), state, and federal level. Plus, a legal due diligence report will also search for any state and federal tax proceedings against the company.

Most businesses with more than five or ten years of operating history will have been involved in a civil court case of some kind. Dental practices even more so, because of the likelihood of a malpractice suit, legitimate or not. There is no rule for quantifying exactly how many legal cases could be considered as normal; however, you should consult with your valuation company once you have a report of the history of legal proceedings. The valuation expert can help you compare your dental practice with others. In some ways, a legal review comes down to common sense. If you see a history that includes more than two workplace related cases (harassment, stress, etc.), several malpractice suits, and ongoing tax problems, you should reconsider buying into the practice. A history of legal problems will also give you some significant leverage when negotiating the buy-in price. If you are buying into a practice with a poor history of legal proceedings, you should expect those problems to continue, therefore seriously putting future profits at risk.

Partner Due Diligence

If you want to know more about each person who is currently a partner in the practice, you will likely have to perform a discreet background check. The partners are not likely to agree for you to review their personal lives, and may take serious offence at the prospect. However, investigating the personal history of future business partners is very common. And it's a responsible move for you.

Again, this will require the work of a private investigator. Because most court cases are publicly available, you will be able to see each individual's history of legal problems. In addition, you will get an idea of any tax problems and bankruptcy proceedings.

Don't be shocked when you see that your future business partners have had their share of legal tangles. Most people have been part of a marital, financial, medical, or other civil case. Lawsuits are difficult to avoid. You should be focusing on any criminal cases or excessive civil proceedings. (Also don't be shocked if one of the partners has a DUI. They are more common than you might think.) Again, there is no way to quantify what is a reasonable legal history. This is a judgment call; you will be in business with these partners. You have to be comfortable with their history, knowing it is something of an indication of their future behavior.

If you have to bring up a concern over the legal history of one of the partners, do it discreetly. Although you can probably use the information to push down the buy-in price, a mishandling of the information could mean that the practice pulls the buy-in offer altogether, along with your current position as an employed dentist. At a minimum, it could create an uncomfortable working environment for you as a new partner.

Letter of Intent:

Once you have a completed practice valuation, and once you have reviewed any additional investigations that could impact the valuation, you and your lawyer will prepare a Letter of Intent (LOI). The LOI is not a legal contract; the LOI is an indication to the dental practice that you are serious about buying into the business.

The letter of intent is not a lengthy document; it's a letter. The letter briefly outlines the key points of your offer to buy into the practice, including your initial financial offer. The LOI is simply a first step, and generally, there is nothing binding if the practice accepts the letter and negotiations begin.

If the practice had been reviewing several potential candidates for partnership, you will want to generate a LOI quickly. Don't delay in acquiring an unbiased valuation and investigative reports. Then, you can use the LOI to demand that the practice cease negotiations with any other candidates. Acting quickly can help you eliminate your competition. If the negotiations with you fall apart and you and the practice don't sign a contract, then you can issue an additional letter withdrawing your offer and freeing the practice to start negotiating with other candidates.

You will have to decide upon a figure for your initial financial offer for the LOI. Most business owners over-estimate the value of their own businesses; especially those who don't frequently review how a business is evaluated. If your investigations have given you a reason to offer substantially less than what the valuation indicates, you and your lawyer will have to briefly explain in the letter why your offer is so low. If the practice hasn't added a partner in the last decade, you might find that the current partners experience a certain degree of shock at your offer.

If the practice owners scoff at your offer, don't panic. By the time you and your lawyer create an LOI, you should have a firm understanding of the business's value. The current partners, however, may not have done their due diligence to determine how much to expect. In fact, the current partners may have simply landed on their own price for a buy-in based on an arbitrary need, like the cost of a new x-ray machine or the price for buying a permanent office. With the effort you've put forth to create the LOI, you might be walking into the negotiations as the savviest businessperson in the room. And if your offer is based upon sound calculations, then you should feel confident standing by it.

Legal Entities That Protect You.

Deciding to start a practice also involves knowing the type of legal entity that you want to choose to create. There are a few options for practice owners.

The first option is to do nothing and simply remain a sole proprietor. A sole proprietor is someone who owns an unincorporated business without any partners. For instance, a dentist graduates from dental school, goes to work as an associate at someone's practice, and then one day decides to become a practice owner. The dentist opens up the office and doesn't do anything else. While it might sound simple (and simple often means good), these days, it is one of the worst ways to be a practice owner because you don't get any of the protection of a corporation or an LLC, depending on your state, and the structure of a general or limited partnership.

Basically, as soon as you are earning some revenue, you are in business as a sole proprietor. At the beginning, there are no state filings, but also there is no separation between the assets of the business and those of the owner. Since business and personal becomes all one thing, your personal assets can be used to satisfy any eventual business debts and liabilities. In other words, being a sole proprietor can put your personal assets at risk.

Now, there are some advantages. A sole proprietorship is obviously easy to create because there is nothing to file. There is no state paperwork because there is no state filing. Since you don't have any entities to file, there is no separate tax filing. All business income or losses are filed on your personal return. That is not a good thing from an audit perspective. In our experience, sole proprietors get audited more frequently as compared to corporations, but the lack of separate tax filings can be considered an advantage. There are no other corporate formalities either, so there are some advantages, but not enough to overcome deciding to become a sole proprietor versus an LLC or a corporation.

We feel very strongly about sole proprietorships and believe that no young dentist owning a practice should be a sole proprietor. In previous generations, many dentists were advised not to turn their business into a corporation for various reasons, but that is not really the recommendation anymore. Any strong CPA will advise a dentist to become a corporation, an LLC, or some other type of legal entity allowed by their specific state.

The second, and preferred option, is to consider classifying your business as a professional corporation - and these corporations can be opened in almost every state. Many business owners start this decision making process by thinking about the taxation differences between the two different kinds of corporations: an S-corporation ("S-Corp") or a C-corporation ("C-Corp"). An S-Corp is something called a 'pass-through tax entity', which is very similar to a limited liability company (LLC). A C-Corp gets taxed as a separate entity. Basically, that means that owning a C-Corp involves double taxation at the corporate level and when the profits are distributed to the shareholder (i.e., the dentist) in the form of a dividend.

Generally speaking, almost all of our clients pick an S-Corp over a C-Corp because they don't want to be taxed twice – an S-Corp means more money in their pocket. The second reason is usually because a C-Corp is only appropriate if you're receiving private equity money and if you have more than 20 shareholders, which is why the Microsoft and the Googles of the world become C-Corps. Most professionals, obviously including dentists, become S-Corps because of those advantages.

Some states allow for a professional to be an LLC or a PLLC. An LLC protects its members (similar to shareholders) from personal liability, which will be reviewed later in detail. An LLC allows for more flexibility in management than with a corporation, because corporations have certain set structures; directors will oversee the business decisions while officers are responsible for other aspects of running the business. An LLC does not have that same built-in formality. In most corporations, the dentist has all of those roles (so it's not as bad as it sounds), but there are some corporate formalities. Another benefit of the LLC is that its 'pass-through taxation' means that taxes are not paid at the business level, as would happen with a C-Corp. With an LLC, the taxes are recorded in the personal return, but are only paid on an individual level. In other words, you are taxed individually on how much you earn from your practice.

While LLCs and corporations sound very similar, there are some key differences between them. The biggest difference is that certain states simply do not allow owners to create an LLC. For example, in California a dentist cannot own a dental practice through an LLC; the company must be a corporation. In other states, the rules are different. A dental practice can be operated through an LLC, although sometimes these LLCs go by the title of Professional LLC (PLLC). That sort of information should always be checked at the earliest stages of seeking to own a practice, because learning this information should be considered a number one priority.

You may have noticed that you can now find online companies which will "help you" to incorporate your business. But you should be wary of going this route. One of the reasons why our company always counsels against people using a web service for business incorporation is because they don't differentiate between professional dentists and other businesses - for example, a dry cleaning shop or a coffee shop can be an LLC. And you shouldn't fall for claims that these services can be "specialized" to help you. Our dentists will even call these web service companies and state what they are doing and what type of business they are seeking to form, thinking they are getting good advice, but they are really getting *bad* advice because web service operators are not trained properly; they are not lawyers and usually are not familiar with the specific dental board rules governing dental professional corporations. Once the web service incorporates the dentists as LLCs, those dentists have just violated a number of rules enacted by dental boards throughout the United States.

Another difference between LLCs and corporations pertains to business losses. Both corporations and S-Corps allow owners to use business losses on their personal tax returns as deductions if you have a good CPA, and that's a huge advantage for those beginning a start-up and buying a practice, for example. There are also certain advantages in terms of self-employment, Social Security, and Medicare taxes as an S-Corp that are not available to an owner of an LLC. Owners can also offset some non-business income with losses from the business - so, again, huge advantage.

Finally, while there are sometimes ownership restrictions when it comes to choosing your incorporation route, usually this is not an issue in dentistry. An S-Corp can have no more than 100 owners, but that is rarely something that is going to happen anyway, at least not with the majority of our clients. One issue is that owners cannot be non-resident aliens. To own a corporation in the United States, you need to be a resident alien or citizen, but you can't be a non-resident alien. An S-Corp cannot be owned by another C-Corp or LLC either.

Three Solid Reasons to Either File as a Corporation or an LLC (as opposed to a Sole Proprietorship)

So we're already touched on this a bit, but the Corporation vs. Sole Proprietorship issue is an important enough one to revisit in more detail.

The first reason to choose a corporation is because you can enjoy limited liability which means that if you are sued then your personal assets are protected from creditors or plaintiffs. It is important to note that malpractice is not covered by the limited liability protection that incorporation provides, so it's vital to have sufficient coverage.

Second, you get some tax benefits with self-employment taxes. There are legal tax-saving games that the IRS allows owners to play with Social Security and Medicare taxes. Most of our dentists can save between $5,000 and $12,000 on average, which is nothing to sneeze at, just by engaging in simple strategies. If your CPA doesn't know what to do, then it's time to change.

The third reason is something you'll hear nowhere else but from me. Follow this link, **www.StrategicDentists.com** and we will send you a summary of that third option.

There are two typical drawbacks commonly mentioned for corporations. One, the owner usually has to pay their state an annual fee for the privilege of being incorporated in that state. The second drawback is having to pay a CPA to file a tax return for your corporation. Even though you're not paying taxes with your S-Corp, it is flowing through and passing to you personally, so you do have to file an informational tax return every year.

We usually suggest that practice owners set aside an annual budget of $2,000 for being incorporated. But if you have a strong CPA, you'll be able to save much more than that so as to make these additional expenses inconsequential.

Limited Partnerships and Annual Obligations

The last option in terms of classification of your business is to turn the business into a partnership. If you want to start your practice with two or more people, you can be a partnership. Most states do not allow limited partnerships for dentists, but you can be a general partnership, which either means that two legal entities or two individual people are getting into business with one another.

There's no limited liability with a partnership by itself, but we always recommend to dentists to incorporate themselves as an S-Corp, so your corporation enters into a partnership with your partner's corporation; that means you also have limited liability at that level, while retaining the perks of being a corporation.

The Lease

Whether you are opening a practice from scratch or purchasing one, the lease will be one of the most important documents you will sign. We have discussed leases generally throughout this book, but we will now get into more details about the lease itself, so that you can be certain you understand the relevant terms and what they could mean for your practice. There are three types of leases that are most common.

The first kind of lease is a Triple Net Lease (NNN). If you see a flyer that says '$2.00 sq./ft. NNN', that means it's a Triple Net lease. This is the most common type of lease available and, as you might expect, it is the worst kind of lease in the market. It is the worst kind of lease because the tenant (you) will pay for your pro-rata portion of taxes, insurance, maintenance, common areas, such as the parking lot, the lobby, the elevators, and the roof. This can increase the cost of your lease very significantly.

When a landlord says, "This space is $2 a square foot, triple net," your first question should be, "How much per square foot is the triple net?" If they say another 90 cents, then your rent is really $2.90 rather than $2.00. They combine those numbers on a month-to-month basis. Around the country, the average is somewhere between 40 to 65 cents, though big high-rise buildings will be much higher. Smaller buildings without a great expanse of common area will not include a lot of expenses, so the rent will be lower.

The second type of lease is a Full-Service Lease. Basically when the terms state '$2.00 sq./ft., full service', that means the renter (you) will pay $2.00 per square foot but nothing else. You will not pay for taxes, common areas, or any of those related items. It is just $2 per square foot. Although it is the best kind of lease to have, as you can imagine, it is also the least common because landlords want to pass on those costs to you. Usually, general office buildings have full service for professional office users like law firms or CPA firms. Usually, commercial spaces, retail shops, shopping centers, or medical/dental buildings are offered Triple Net leases.

The third type of lease is a Base Year Lease. It goes by a lot of different names, but these hybrid leases have traits of a Triple Net and Full Service lease. Essentially, you pay both your rent and the difference between a base year and the year the expense was recognized.

So for example, let's say the year is 2016 and the leasing is $2.00 sq./t Base Year. That means if you open your office in 2016, you will not pay any other expense other than $2.00 sq./ft. because your base year is 2016. Say in 2017, the cost of managing the building increased $1.00 sq./ft. a square foot and you occupied 10% of that. If the cost of building management increased $1.00 sq./ft. a square foot and you occupy 10% of the area, you will pay $2.00 sq./ft. on your base rent plus 10 cents, which is your pro-rata portion of the increase from the base year of the expense.

These are good leases and a great alternative to Triple Net Leases. In terms of securing any type of lease, do your homework, and remember that the importance of securing a beneficial lease will only increase over time - this is why you want to get the best lease that you can the first time around.

Lease Negotiations Process

The lease negotiations process really starts with something called a letter of intent (LOI). The LOI is a way for you, and hopefully a commercial broker working with you, to summarize the business terms that you want to propose to the landlord to lease a space. Sometimes landlords will give you a draft of an LOI and tell you to add the rest, and sometimes they will ask you to just put it together yourself.

1. The Letter of Intent (LOI): This letter consists of the lease terms, i.e. the length of time that you want the term to be and payment terms. Usually, a minimum term length is ten years, especially if you're starting a practice from scratch, but our firm has seen five years with some options. There are two five-year options or three five-year options, but the most typical term is ten years with two five-year options.t Most lenders require at least a ten-year loan when they finance a startup or acquisition transaction. While this length of time is pretty typical in the business world, it can sometimes sound strange to a young dentist who may have only executed personal leases on apartments before, for example, and for whom one year sounds like a typical lease term. Knowing what terms should and should not surprise you is one benefit to using a commercial realtor during this process.

2. The Rent: Determining when to pay the rent and how much that rent should be is not as easy as it sounds. If you are using a commercial broker, he or she will be able to do a market study to determine

the fair market value of the area, and also to advise you on what is considered a standard annual increase. On average, rents increase either based on a flat percentage, such as 3%, or it is tied to the consumer price index which is a function of inflation.

If you're starting a practice from scratch, you need to find out the date when your rent will start. It should not start on the day that you signed the lease because you still have to do some construction, which most landlords understand. However, the skill of your negotiations will dictate the amount of "free rent" you can get before starting the rent payments (meaning the amount of time that you can be in the building without paying rent - such as during the construction process). The longer this time period is, the better. We recommend trying to get 6-9 months of free rent from the time you execute your lease, or 3 months from the time you receive your certificate of occupancy. Please keep in mind that these are recommendations and that the local market dynamics of supply and demand really impact how much landlords give in when negotiating leases. If you are purchasing a practice, negotiating a reduction in rent from a landlord is very difficult because typically the landlord already has a committed tenant in the seller. They will, however, negotiate extensions or some sort of lease assignment.

3. Security Deposits: All landlords will ask for a security deposit, usually one to two months' worth of your rent. Don't be taken aback by that amount, but anything more than that should be negotiated down. With one of our recent clients, the landlord

asked for five months' worth of a security deposit, which was ridiculous, but usually, the requested amount is one to two months.

4. Repair Costs: When reviewing a lease, it is important to pay close attention to who pays for repair costs. Usually, everything inside your space is your responsibility, and everything outside of your space, where you don't have control, is usually the landlord's responsibility. But it is important to note who is responsible for repairing glass windows or HVAC units, providing for appropriate gardening and landscaping on the premises, or updating common area light fixtures.

5. Improvements and Alterations: Obviously, it is important to get an idea of the type of limitations, if any, your landlord will put on the improvements of the space or any future alterations. If you are buying a practice and you want to move a wall or change the paint color, those are things to discuss. If you are starting a practice from scratch, obviously the improvement part is very important because you are building a practice from nothing. For startups, we recommend that you have your preliminary design ready for the landlord to approve before lease execution or add reasonableness language so that he cannot deny your design.

6. Paying for Construction: If you are starting a practice from scratch, you will have to do a lot of construction. As a result, you will have to negotiate with the landlord in terms of who will pay for which items and whether they will give you any money for tenant improvements. Some landlords will offer some cash to build your office; sometimes it's good to get that cash and sometimes it's not because the money is not actually *free*, of course.

When a landlord provides tenant improvement dollars, they are usually loaning you the money by increasing your rent. That is a terrible loan because you end up paying for that loan throughout the term of your lease and it will continue to go up exponentially. For instance, if the landlord gives you $20.00 sq./ft. for 2000 sq./ft. office for a grand total of $40,000, but then increases your rent by around $0.25 a sq./ft., you will end up paying $60,000 in rent you shouldn't have paid over the first 10 years (assuming no annual rent increase) and $120,000 over 20 years (again, assuming no annual rent increase). If you add the typical 3% yearly rent increase, then the amount you pay the landlord in exchange for that $40,000 "free money" ends up being astronomical. Many times we recommend that dentists simply get more money from a lender instead of getting money from the landlord. This is a tricky negotiation, so it is important to have some professionals involved.

7. <u>Exclusivity</u>. You have to negotiate the kind of use you want for your space. You might initially want to just put down 'dentistry', but you may not want that forever. If you're very entrepreneurial as a general dentist, you may want to just put down 'general dentistry' so that you can have a pediatric dentist next to you; maybe an orthodontist will open up next door so you can all cross-refer patients to each other. Together, when those three types are in close proximity to each other (general dentist, pediatric dentist, and orthodontist), this has proven to be a very successful business model for a lot of our clients and have allowed them to provides a lot of cross-referrals. You need to think about these possibilities well in advance so that you can incorporate your goals into your lease negotiations.

8. Sub-Letting: The assignment provisions of any lease are very important. It is very important to review those provisions allowing you to transfer your interest in the lease regardless of your age. You might think that you won't have to worry about this issue because you will be working for the next 25 to 30 years, but accidents do happen - disability happens. Things happen that can cause you to change your mind and sell your practice without any fault of your own, it's just life; you've got to be able to assign or sub-let the premises to someone else.

9. Default Provision. You need to carefully review this section of your lease and determine which events will cause you to be in default. For example, if you're traveling and your rent is three days late because the bank holiday fell on the due date, is that a default? Can the landlord take back the space or cause other problems for your practice? You don't want to give the landlord any reason to impact your ability to be an owner or stay in that facility just because of a small error or default.

10. Options to Renew: Obviously, you want to get as many options to renew as possible. Options are to your advantage because they belong to you, not to the landlord. If you're lucky enough to have a ten-year lease, by the tenth year or sooner, perhaps you will have outgrown the space or now you are planning to buy a space so you don't have to renew your lease option. On the other hand, if you're happy where you are, and surrounding rent prices are rocketing through the roof, then you may want to exercise your option and stay there. As I mentioned earlier, a ten-year lease with two five-year options is usually ideal for a start-up. For

someone buying a practice, it all depends on the location and your growth plan (an issue which will be covered later on in this book).

Misconceptions and Other Important Lease Topics

One common misconception with an LOI is that it can just be signed and still leave an opportunity to renegotiate the terms at some later point. This is a major error and something you never want to do. Even though an LOI is not binding, which means you can walk away from the transaction (no harm no foul), you do not get to renegotiate the LOI once it has been signed unless something drastically changes. For instance, if the landlord states that you will get access to 10,000 square feet and ten parking spaces, but after viewing the space, you find out it's 1,500 square feet with one parking space - this would be considered a drastic change. You never want to just sign an LOI because landlords get really upset if you try to change any terms.

The good news is that leases are usually very negotiable. Even if you are in a high-demand area, we find that landlords are usually willing to negotiate because they love your "youth," for lack of a better term. They love young dentists because they know you will be there long-term, you pay your rent on time, and you will be successful. It is important to always negotiate, but always do it with a professional, with your commercial broker on the economic terms and then with a lawyer on the rest. You may want to work with a lawyer from the very beginning to make sure that you don't give anything away. There are strategies that can be put in place to get you the best deal, both on rent and other components of the lease.

You do have to know who is representing you, so I always counsel against working with a dual broker. This is because the landlord's broker works for the landlord, of course. Even if they say, "Oh, I can work with you," it's always a bad idea because their interests lie with the landlord who will get them more business than you as a renter, who will probably never lease again because you will be in that location for a long time. This should help to explain where the landlord's broker's loyalties will lie. Find your own broker or, if you've already started discussions with a landlord, hire an attorney to help you. Each side should have his or her own representative.

As for rent, it is usually discussed at a per square footage rate and is set on a monthly basis. Sometimes you'll see a very large number, for example '$24 a square foot'. That means it's $24 per square foot per year (12 months), which comes out to $2 per square foot per month. The same thing applies if the terms state $36 a square foot or $3 a foot. A lot of brokers will list it per month, so they'll say it's $2 per square foot. The average rental increase is about 3% per year, year over year, so you need to think about inflation. Sometimes the increase will be spelled out as a flat number, like 2% to 4%; sometimes an extreme increase will reach as high as 5%, but it should really stay between the 2% to 4% range.

Sometimes, instead of using a flat number, inflation will be based on something called the CPI (Consumer Price Index). Every metropolitan area has a CPI, which is really a measure of inflation. It is not super complex to figure out because it gets published every month, but it is something to review and determine the expected amount of increase in your rent. When the economy is down, CPI is great, because it's sometimes close to zero or a negative number. But during normal years it's usually regarded as close to 3%, so you shouldn't see a huge difference either way.

Sharing Real Estate Taxes and Common Area Maintenance (CAM): A landlord may require a tenant to pay for real estate taxes in many different ways. In a Triple Net lease, the landlord requires a tenant to pay their entire pro-rata share of it, or the landlord may agree to a certain base. Then you would pay for the pro-rata portion of any increase over the base amount as previously mentioned. This is also very true with CAM. In an office with condominiums and other tenants, you pay your pro-rata share of all of the CAM fees.

Grace Period: Be sure to specify a grace period in your lease. Checks do get lost in the mail, and people do go on vacation. The landlord should not be able to just assess a late fee, or in a worst-case scenario (which I have sometimes seen), terminate a lease if payment is not received on the due date. The reason is because you have invested a lot into the space and it is not to your advantage, so you need to have a grace period. The usual number would be five to 20 days, but typically it is closer to five days.

Option to Buy: If you have the ability with a smaller building or some other a building that would be affordable, you definitely want to add an option to buy or a right of first refusal. Some landlords are willing to grant renters the option to buy or the right of first refusal if the property is sold. Out of thousands of clients nationwide, not one of them has regretted owning a building. That's partly because of the process we take them through; we show them the advantages and how the numbers align with their strategic goals. The other part is that it is always better to own your own building and build some equity into the property as opposed to paying just rent. Options to buy are absolutely great and should be sought whenever possible.

Sub-Leasing: In the actual lease document itself, you want to outline the right to be able to sub-let to specialists or others. There is some language that you also need to review, called the 'duty to mitigate'. In case you have to leave the premises, it's important that the landlord should have a duty to rent it immediately. There is a legal obligation to do this already, but it is nice to state it in the lease because landlords are sometimes slow to find new renters.

A Personal Guarantee: It is not uncommon for a landlord to require you, as a dentist, to sign a personal guarantee. If you are married, my strategic advice is to avoid having your spouse sign the personal guarantee. The best landlords will have the dentist and their spouse sign the guarantee due to the way that some states' property rights are set up. Various states offer almost no recourse for a landlord unless they get the spouse to also sign the personal guarantee. If you can, definitely try to avoid this requirement.

Burn-Off or De-Escalation Period: This is something that our firm highly recommends and does quite frequently, called a 'burn-off period' or a 'de-escalation period'. This basically means that the personal guarantee goes away after a certain amount of time, say from two to four years.

Landlords are very hesitant to do this but our success rate is about 40%, so it is worth trying. Many lawyers and brokers will push back or tell you not to include it, but we highly, highly recommend it.

Human Resources: The Silent Killer

As an owner, you need to know how to hire employees. Obviously, human resources (HR) rules apply whether you buy a practice or start one from scratch. And most legal problems start with the most basic HR laws.

In fact, it is believed that HR lawsuits are now outpacing malpractice lawsuits against dentists.

For example, the questions you can ask in interviews or when you are about to hire an employee can be tricky because there are some questions that you can ask and some questions that you should not ask.

Questions related to the following are always off limits:

- Race

- Religion (although you may ask if a person is able to work weekends, if such an inquiry is necessary)

- Age (other than verifying that an employee is 18 years of age or older)

- Country of origin (although you may verify proof of legal right to work upon hire)

- Disability (you may ask if the applicant is able to perform the requirements of the job)

- Political affiliations

- Sexual orientation

- Gender (meaning that you cannot make presumptions as to whether someone is capable of performing a job based upon his or her gender

- Family status (whether someone is married, has children, etc.)

In addition to the above, it is also a good idea to avoid asking too many personal questions, especially anything related to someone's financial status, housing neighborhood, etc. We understand that this may make your interview process feel overly "formalized" or impersonal, but the bottom line is that you have to protect your business in all aspects. While you want to find the right person to hire for your position, you should never put your business at risk while doing so.

These are examples of the questions that you can ask potential employees:

- Tell us why you're interested in this job.

- Describe your ideal work environment.

- Do you prefer a job with clearly defined tasks or one that's more self-directed?

- What excites you about this position and what do you think would be a stretch for you?

- What would you do if the owner asked you to do something that a manager or another employee asked you not to do?

- What type of relationship do you feel you have with your current manager or supervisor?

- Give me an example of how you think outside of the box?

- How do you handle stress?

Those are good questions to ask because they are allowed.

Here are some examples of the questions that you cannot ask potential employees:

- Do you own or rent your home?
- When did you graduate high school?
- What religious days do you observe?
- Do you belong to any organizations or clubs?
- Where did you grow up?
- Do you have any children?
- Where did you serve in the military?
- What is your nationality?

For additional information on questions you can and cannot ask applicants and employees, please visit our website at www.strategicdentists.com.

Many of our clients use social media for hiring, but you have to be really careful about using social media in hiring (Facebook, Twitter, Instagram, etc.); you may see things that you are not allowed to see about an employee or things that might leave the impression that you discriminated against them by race or religion just by looking them up. We highly recommend that you don't Google them or use social media to access that information because it can all cause trouble. If you are going to do it, we ask that you do it yourself and don't tell anybody; definitely don't delegate that task to somebody else.

The next step is to determine how to hire employees and the foundation of compliance begins with the new hire documentation. In most states, you need from five to 18 documents, depending on your particular state, for each and every employee, to cover necessary requirements. These include many federal and state mandated documents and in certain jurisdictions there are local requirements that must be met.

The next important item for HR compliance is an employee manual, which is a handbook for all of your employees. A handbook details all of the rules of your office such as what time the office opens and morning huddle meeting times, disciplinary procedures, details about vacation or other benefits and dress code. Drafting a handbook is an art because you don't want it to have so much detail that you cannot follow your own rules but you don't want it to be superficial and unclear.

Also, when we talk to the plaintiff lawyers who sue our dentists, they tell us that an employment manual is very important to them. If one does not exist, then they consider the lawsuit as the proverbial low-hanging fruit. The best practice in this area is to get an employment handbook and to update it every year. Some great resources like HR for Health will update it for free as part of their service for you.

As an analogy, an employee handbook is like a toothbrush. You don't want to use another person's toothbrush, but you must have one. Also, you've got to know how to use it, how often to use it, and the kind of toothbrush matters. It is not necessary to spend $2,000 or $3,000 on a lawyer or an HR company to put it together for you, and we highly recommend that you don't get one from your payroll company. We recommend HR for Health because they provide a complimentary customized handbook as part of their software and it is updated every year for you.

It is also important to know when to provide lunch and breaks to your employees and also to whom you have to pay overtime. These items fall under the category of Wage & Hour and it is the single largest category of claims filed against dentists.

So make sure you get some professional advice from HR for Health in this area and don't assume that the previous owner or your current employer is handling their HR requirements correctly.

Insurance Policies

Finally, you need to contact your insurance broker to acquire various types of insurance regardless of whether you're starting a practice from scratch or purchasing a practice.

For talking points, you will want to discuss these topics with your insurance broker about your policies: names of the protected parties, the coverage limits, the exclusions, and some of the conditions.

As a primer for that conversation, here is some general information about insurance:

The first type of insurance is professional liability coverage. There are claims-made insurance and occurrence insurance. Claims-made policies pay claims reported to the insurer during the term of the policy or within a specific term after the policy expires. Premiums usually rise step by step for a few years; as your risk increases, the policy amount goes up, but then at some point it matures and no longer rises as much as it was doing for the first few years. An occurrence policy pays claims arising from incidents that occur during the policy term, no matter when the claim is reported to the insurer. These usually cost a lot more because of the way the insurance company calculates risk, but it is usually regarded as being a more protective policy than the other.

The second category of insurance relevant to your practice is business property insurance. This protects the physical assets of the practice including dental equipment, supplies, and patient charts.

The third category of insurance is general liability. The general liability insurance protects you from claims of injuries such as slips and falls, and the loss or damage of business property.

Fourth, you need automobile insurance if you will have your staff attend lunch-and-learns or take items to referral sources.

Fifth, umbrella liability insurance is always a great insurance to have as a business owner because it protects you from any other problems that are not covered already.

Sixth, you should have overhead insurance, in case you cannot practice anymore for some reason; this insurance covers your overhead. It does not pay your salary, but it covers all of your employee costs and other business expenses like rent.

Seventh, you need worker's compensation insurance ("workers comp") if your practice will hire any employees. It's illegal to not have workers comp - you can be found to be criminally liable with jail time and severe fines - so make sure to get it.

Eighth, if you're in a partnership, you've got to have a buy and sell agreement with life and disability insurance. That protects you and your partner in case one of you passes away.

On top of that, life insurance will also be required by many landlords and by the banks. Many of our clients have life insurance already, but we ask them to get another policy on top of their existing ten-year or twenty-year term, just for the landlord and for the bank.

Steps You Can Take Even If You're Not Yet Ready for Practice Ownership

Many of our clients are new dentists who know that they are interested in pursuing practice ownership in the future, but will not be ready to do so for some time. Most are associates who are looking down the road towards seeking a partnership with their current practice. Others are unsure whether they will want to stay with their current practice or branch out on their own. Regardless of your plan, there are steps that you can take now which will make things easier down the road, when you ARE ready to pursue ownership:

1. Get, or keep, your finances in order. For many young dentists, student loans can be crippling. And when you are trying to start or support a young family, it is not always easy to save money. But to the extent possible, you should add to your savings and maintain financial responsibility. When you are ready to pursue practice ownership, regardless of whether you are buying into, taking over, or starting a new practice, the more of your own money that you can bring to the table when you do so, the better.

2. Be cognizant of the upsides, and downsides, of the practice ownership processes that you are able to witness. For example, let's say that you believe that your current office would be more comfortable for your patients if you provided a television in the waiting room, or Wi-Fi service, different magazine selections, what have you. You

should make note of that information now. If you later decide to open your own practice, then you can incorporate those ideas into your business (making it less likely that you will forget something), or, if you buy into a practice, then you can add those ideas to your list of suggestions or intended changes once you are a partner. These examples are of simple changes, but you should use this approach for any number of ideas which strike you as you are headed towards practice ownership.

3. Start considering potential practice locations. Again, you don't have to start taking any concrete steps towards ownership at this point. But the more research that you do into potential neighborhoods, foot traffic and other demographics, etc., the better position you will be in if you choose to start your own practice in the future.

4. Take advantage of any free time that you have while you have it. For many associates, transitioning into practice ownership requires a significant time investment. Therefore, if you know that you will be pursuing ownership in the future, then you should take advantage of any free time that you have now, while you can. Consider longer family vacations, etc. - and it is good to acknowledge with your family and/or friends that you may have less free time in the future and therefore wish to enjoy that time right now.

The bottom line is that it is never too early to prepare for practice ownership. Many dentists wait until they are ready to move forward with ownership before realizing that they know little about the business end of owning a dental practice. The more you educate yourself now, the better you'll be once the time comes and you are ready to own your own practice.

How to Prepare to Start a Practice in 30 days

The decision whether to start your own dental practice is a serious one. It requires preparation, and a dedication of both your time and resources. There are difficult analyses and choices to be made, and it is not a task, which should be taken on lightly.

That being said, it is possible to start a dental practice in a short amount of time, if you are willing to do everything it takes to make your practice happen. If you are serious about starting your own business but you are concerned about how long such an endeavor may take, I am here to tell you that it *can* be done but you need to take the first steps, which seem to always be the most difficult.

This leads us to the most important component of getting started on opening a dental practice in 30 days: Your mindset.

If you have been thinking about opening a practice for some time, then you may have already made up your mind as to your preferred location, practice type, practice atmosphere, type of online presence, etc. But if you have not made some of those decisions, then you must be prepared to do so, and to do so quickly. And you will not be able to afford spending time questioning your choices. Once you decide upon a location, then you must stop wasting time looking at other possibilities. The same is true for equipment, employees, etc. If you are someone who is often indecisive, then you must overcome this trait or accept that your purchase process may take longer than you hope. There is no "right" way to open a practice, and there is nothing wrong with shopping around and taking your time to make important decisions related to your business. However, when it comes to starting a practice, the first 30 days is important and quick decision-making is required.

Quick decision-making doesn't mean it's rushed or not deliberate. It simply means that you perform research and rely on that research and trusted advisers to make decisions that have a low-risk profile and a history of high success.

Finally, while preparing yourself to start a practice within 30 days is definitely possible, you should go into this process with the understanding that there may be circumstances beyond your control, which may cause delays. Maybe your prospective landlord has to leave town for an emergency and cannot execute your lease in your preferred timeframe. Maybe you have problems filling an essential role in your practice due to a lack of applicants. Maybe your lender has a last-minute request for documentation that will take time to produce. The bottom line is that delays happen, and that you cannot control every aspect of this process. But if you can approach this task with the correct mindset, and you do everything within your control to make it happen as quickly as possible, then you will have laid the groundwork for a very short path to practice ownership.

If you are interested in preparing to open a dental practice within 30 days, below are some suggested steps to follow. This list is not exhaustive - it is simply intended to serve as a guideline for addressing all requirements necessary for starting a practice in a short amount of time. Some of these steps may require more or less time, depending upon your location and needs.

Week One
Days 1-3: Decide Upon a Location

As stated above, choosing a location is one of the most important decisions that you will make when starting a practice. If you are looking to start a practice, then the best decision that you can make during this step of the process is to hire a professional to lighten your load. Hiring a commercial broker to provide you with some location possibilities can reduce the amount of legwork that you have to put into the process. Make sure that your broker is aware of your desired timeframe, and confirm that the broker is not too busy with other projects to make a lot of his/her time available to you right away. If you are looking for a broker, simply give us a call and we would be happy to refer you to some wonderful people.

As for the location itself, we recommend picking one or two cities where the commercial broker can focus their attention. And it is important to remember that there is never a perfect location so be ready to make some concessions if you wish to start your practice right away. Choosing a location, which is already set up for a dental practice, for example, might be a great decision to limit costs when you are first starting.

Days 3-4: Choose your Dental Attorney for the Lease Negotiations

Once you have picked a location, you can begin lease negotiations. The lease negotiation process is another step in which seeking professional help is a great idea. If you do not yet have an attorney to assist you with this process, then this is a good time to hire one.

The commercial broker can negotiate the business terms of the lease on your behalf, but your attorney will review the legal language to make sure that you are not putting yourself at risk. By outsourcing these steps to specialists, you free up your time to work on other steps of the process, and you can rely upon the fact that your interests are being protected. Of course, no final decisions should be made without your input, but you should leave the details to the broker and attorney to the extent possible.

Note, however, that the decisions, which are made at this point in, the process have the potential to affect your practice for years to come. Do not allow your desire to open a practice quickly override your good sense. If you do not feel that a lease term is fair, or if you think that it will put you into a bad position in the future, then you should not concede this point simply so that you can open your doors sooner. Remember that while you are seeking a quick turnaround on the lease, you can potentially be causing yourself a lot of future headaches if the negotiation process is not completed thoroughly and correctly the first time around.

Finally, while you should be negotiating lease terms after you have found a location and negotiated a letter of intent, you should not enter into any binding agreements until you have secured financing for your business - which leads us to our next topic.

Days 5-6: Determine Your Financial Needs and speak to 2 Lenders

Now that you have begun the lease negotiation process, you should have some idea of the finances that starting and running your business will require. At this stage, it is important to begin analyzing your financial situation, so that you can begin to determine how much you have on hand, how much you will need to borrow, and what options you have for borrowing. Gather your financial records and prepare yourself to tackle the money end of your practice.

Days 6-7: Choose a Corporate Structure

The details of the various available corporate structures are discussed in the book, and all of those same details apply when you are seeking to open a practice right away. Review your options, decide upon a corporate structure, and meet with your attorney to complete and file all of the necessary paperwork to make your chosen structure legal.

Week Two

Day 8: Begin Financing Process

You will begin to see that many steps of this 30-day process are related to the financial end of your business, and for good reason. Just as with your lease, you want to complete this process quickly, but you do not want to be careless. This stage should be spent deciding upon a lender by comparing potential rates and lending structures. If you are fortunate enough to have all of the necessary financing on hand, then this process will be simple. But for most dentists, the assistance of a lender will be necessary.

Also, if you plan to borrow part or all of your necessary financing from friends or family members (a route which is not always optimal and which is discussed in more detail in the book), then you should spend this day having your attorney draft a lending/payment agreement between you and the kind soul who is loaning you funds. Just because your lender is a person, and not a bank, does not mean that you should skip out on executing relevant paperwork to protect both of your interests.

Days 9-10: Begin Drafting Your Business Plan

Take your time and be thorough about your needs and goals. If you have already spoken to banks about potential financing, then they may have advised you as to any specifics that they would want in a business plan. If not, then you should use a template for guidance, to make sure that your business plan covers all of your bases and puts you in the best position for securing financing and getting your business started on the right foot.

Day 11: Decide Upon a Lender

Now that you have reviewed potential interest rates and loan structures and you have outlined your needs in a business plan, you can decide which lender is right for you. If you have an established history with a bank, then choosing that same lender may be your best route. The good news is that most commercial lending institutions consider dental practices to be a sound investment; therefore, you should have a few institutions that you are able to choose from, and you are in a good position to negotiate the terms and rate that you prefer. If you have credit issues, however, then your list of potential lenders may be more limited.

Days 12-14: Complete Financing Applications

Once you have chosen a lender, you can begin to complete the necessary applications, which will require you to provide supporting financial documentation. The supporting documentation part of the process will be simplified if you started to gather the information you need during days 5-6. If you did not do so, or if you are having trouble, then you may wish to enlist the help of a CPA at this point. Hiring a CPA is a good idea anyway, since you are likely to need one once your practice is up and running. When submitting your financing applications, it is advisable to let the bank know about your desired timeframe so that they know that you are expecting a quick response and would appreciate their assistance in making this process as simple as possible.

Week Three

Day 15: Determine Payment Structures

At this stage, when we talk about "payment structures," we are talking about how your practice is going to make money. What types of insurance will you accept? Will you provide credit options? How much will you charge for services? Optimally, you would have considered these issues when you were drafting your business plan. But at this point, you will need to start taking steps towards ensuring that your practice is able to follow your envisioned financial routes. You should investigate what you need to do to establish relationships with insurance carriers and credit companies, so as to give yourself, and your future clients, as many financial options as possible.

Day 16: Secure Insurance

Now that you are on the road towards practice ownership, it is time to start protecting your investment. Again, you need to seek the assistance of a professional - here, an insurance broker. Refer to the Insurance section of the book for a more detailed discussion of the types of insurance that you will need to purchase.

Day 17: Begin Hiring Process

Your employees will soon become the lifeblood of your practice, which is why you need to hire the right people from the very beginning. This part of the process may require some time, but it is not really possible to start the hiring process any sooner than this point, since you need to make sure that you have the financing and location to start a practice which will *need* employees in the first place. But now that those tasks have been addressed, the hiring process can begin.

The first steps of the hiring process are deciding which roles you will need to fill, and how much you are willing to pay. Optimally, you would have considered these issues when you were completing your business plan, but it is possible that you may not have been able to make those decisions until you were confident in your financing. Either way, those decisions need to be made now, before you start making your positions available to applicants.

Next, you need to find a way to locate potential employees. Given your timeframe, online advertising of your available positions is likely to get you the fastest responses. Announce your positions on Facebook and/or Twitter, and consider local and national online job search databases.

Keep in mind that you will not want to waste time interviewing applicants who are either unqualified or uninterested in actually working for your practice, so you want to make your job postings as detailed as possible. Your job posting should include the following:

- The title and duties of the position
- The location of your practice (you can just list a general area if your lease paperwork has not yet been finalized)
- Your educational requirements
- The expected work hours, including any potential evening and weekend obligations
- The salary (this is optional, but it may save you time in the long run by limiting your applicant pool to those who are aware of the salary and are comfortable with it)
- The expected start date
- The exact application requirements
- Your contact information, and an explanation as to how application materials should be submitted

By detailing all of the above in your job posting, you can save yourself the time of fielding questions from potential applicants. Also, consider allowing applicants to submit their materials electronically, rather than by mail in order to save time.

You'll note that there is no specific "day" listed here for reviewing applications and conducting interviews. That is because the timeframe of this process will depend heavily on the number and quality of the applications that you receive. Therefore, you will need to fit these components of the hiring process into your schedule over the next two weeks. It is advisable, however, that once you begin receiving applications you review them quickly and set up interviews right away, so that you can begin to staff your practice as quickly as possible.

Day 18: Start Interviewing Equipment Specialists

You cannot run a dental practice without equipment or electrical services, of course. But you should not/cannot begin to order equipment and establish utility services until you have secured your lease and, preferably, your financing. But once you have completed those tasks, you should begin to interview your equipment specialists as they will facilitate and strategize with you on how to and when to order your equipment. As the book explains, it is optimal if you can hire an equipment specialist and possibly an architect to assist you with these processes.

Whether you choose to lease or purchase your equipment, remember to have an attorney review all related paperwork to make sure that they are legally sound and that your assets are protected.

Day 19: Create Business Presence

You likely came up with the name of your practice (even if it is just your personal name) when you decided upon your corporate structure and completed the related paperwork. However, at this point you need to start creating your overall presence. This includes considering a logo (if you wish to use one) and creating and ordering signage, stationery, business cards, etc. Remember that it is easiest to build name recognition if you use the same logo/business name over the course of your practice ownership, so you should decide upon something that you expect to withstand the test of time.

This is also a great time to begin building an online presence. Create a website, Facebook page, twitter account, etc. to get your name out there and to let potential patients know that you will soon be opening a new practice. You do not have to do this yourself, and, in fact, it is advisable that you do not, given your timeframe (even if you possess the necessary skills).

The good news is that creating an online presence is a great, and fast, way to begin advertising. But you should also engage in traditional advertising routes, including local newspapers and signs hung at your location. Make sure that all of your communications include your contact information and expected opening date, and make it clear that you are accepting new patients.

Note that you should create your online presence as soon as possible, so that you can include your website and other social media information in your traditional advertisements. And the more information that you can include on your website (hours of operation, services offered, location, parking, etc.) the better, so that you can reduce the number of phone calls that you have to field from interested potential clients. Also, if you are still engaging in the hiring process, you should include this information on your website and Facebook pages as well, in order to expand your pool of applicants.

Day 20: Select Programs for Accounting, Payroll and Human Resources

If you have never owned a business before, then you may underestimate the importance of purchasing and implementing software for your accounting and payroll needs. These programs, however, are crucial, and will ensure that you are in a good position to be paid, and to pay your employees, as quickly and simply as possible. It is essential that your recordkeeping, both for your clients and for your employees, be in perfect shape from the get-go, so as to avoid putting yourself at unnecessary risk.

Since hiring an HR specialist is not possible for most new practice, HR for Health is an excellent choice to help with everything from employee manuals to tax forms to timecards. They take all of these obligations off of your shoulders, while also ensuring that you are in full compliance with all applicable laws related to sick leave, lunch and rest breaks, and wage requirements (including overtime) for a ridiculously low monthly price. Outsourcing these responsibilities can save you vast amounts of time, money, and headaches.

Day 21: Review progress and follow-up on anything missed from above

This is a good time to begin going through your list of requirements and see what still needs to be addressed. This list is what you will use to tie up all loose ends during week four.

Week Four

Days 22-30: Wrap Everything Up

If you have followed the steps outlined above, then that means that you have taken the initial steps towards completing all tasks necessary as you prepare to start your practice in 30 days. But it is unlikely that you would have been able to start, and finish, all of the above steps in the listed timeframes. Therefore, this is when you need to ensure the completion of each of the above requirements, so that you can open your practice as soon as possible.

So, start at the beginning. Has your lease been finalized? If not, then you need to find out what the holdup is. If there are some small terms, which are preventing the lease completion, then you may have to decide whether you are able to concede on those points to get your lease into effect right away. Hopefully, however, your broker has resolved these issues already and your lease has been put into place, ensuring that you do, in fact, have a place to practice.

Next, if your financing has not gone through and your funds have not yet been issued, then you could have a major problem. If there has been any question as to whether your financing would be approved, then you should not have taken any additional steps before that issue has been resolved. If the problem is that you have been approved but your funds have not yet been released, then you need to see what the issue is. Make it clear that you need those funds to start your business, and that the longer this process takes, the more potential issues you may have ensuring that your business is a success (which, of course, is necessary in order to repay the loan). For most dentists, however, obtaining funds once your loan has been approved is unlikely to be a problem.

Once your funds have been issued, you will likely have to start making payments in order to address the other tasks outlined above. You will need to have funds for rent (with a due date dependent upon the terms of your lease), as well as for equipment, potential utility deposits, advertising, signage, etc. You will also need to make premium payments for your insurance.

In addition to your equipment, you will also need to purchase other items for your office, including furniture, office and restroom supplies, and likely many other small items that you have not yet considered. You will need to purchase magazines (or magazine subscriptions) for your waiting room. You will need to purchase televisions if you are choosing to have cable in your office. It is also highly advisable that you install Wi-Fi for the betterment of your practice and the convenience of your patients.

One way you can minimize your time investment at this stage of the process is to make one of your first hires a flexible front office and back office assistant to whom you can outsource many of these tasks. Remember, however, that even if you have not opened your doors, you cannot hire employees of any type until you have secured all of the necessary tax forms and other documentation required for new employees. You have done all of this work towards opening your practice - you do not want to undo all of those efforts by failing to follow the proper procedures when it comes to hiring employees.

Regardless of whether you outsource or do it yourself, you should be prepared for unexpected expenses to arise during this final time before you officially open your practice. Remember that surprises sometimes (often) come up, and don't allow them to derail you or extinguish your enthusiasm. Starting a practice is quite an accomplishment, and one, which should be celebrated. Take a moment to step back and take pride in your accomplishments.

Now that you know how to prepare yourself to start a practice, you are ready to get started. For your convenience, we have included a handy checklist below to assist you in this process.

If a Dentist Wants to Work with Us

If you are looking to work with us, you can schedule a call or visit the website below to schedule a free strategic call with us. There is no obligation to this call; we discuss your plans and next steps, and how to get to those stated objectives.

At **www.strategicdentists.com**, there is a strategic resource page that describes all the strategic partners with whom we work and who we would highly recommend.

The best way to reach us is to call our office at **925-999-8200**. You can either schedule a time to speak with me directly, or e-mail me at my initials, which is **ao@dmcounsel.com**.

Checklist for Purchasing a Practice

A. Pre planning

- ☐ Pre-qualify with a lender
- ☐ Interview Attorney
- ☐ Interview CPA
- ☐ Interview transition consultants
- ☐ Speak to local practice sale brokers

B. Practice Identified

- ☐ Review practice prospectus
- ☐ Select Attorney
- ☐ Submit letter of intent (LOI)

C. Seller Accepts Your LOI

- ☐ Conduct due diligence with transition consultant or CPA
- ☐ Submit financials to bank
- ☐ Submit credentialing paperwork to insurance companies
- ☐ Submit paperwork for life insurance, disability, malpractice and general liability, among others, to insurance broker
- ☐ Attorney negotiates asset purchase agreement
- ☐ Attorney negotiates lease
- ☐ Establish legal structure

D. Within 30 days of Closing Date

- ☐ Apply for biz license
- ☐ Setup QuickBooks file and bookkeeping structure with CPA
- ☐ Contact HR for Health for new hire employee documents and employee handbook.
- ☐ Submit fictitious business name application
- ☐ Submit applications to dental board

- ☐ Submit oral conscious sedation or general anesthesia permit
- ☐ Open a bank account
- ☐ Draft letter to existing and inactive patients introducing buyer
- ☐ Apply for National Provider Identifier number
- ☐ Begin designing website
- ☐ Design business cards, logo, stationery, etc.

E. Due Diligence in Purchasing a Practice

- ☐ Request tax returns for past 3 years.
- ☐ Request profit & loss statement for last calendar year and year to date
- ☐ Request production and collections reports for past 3 years
- ☐ Request accounts receivables report
- ☐ Request breakdown of procedures for previous year and year to date
- ☐ Request number of new patients for past 3 years
- ☐ Perform chart audit
- ☐ Request adjustment report
- ☐ Request number of hygiene days worked in previous year and year to date
- ☐ Request number of dentist days worked in previous year and year to date
- ☐ Request number of patients seems in the past 6 months, 12 months and 24 months.
- ☐ Request report of what is referred to specialists

Checklist for starting a practice

A. Pre planning

- ☐ Create business plan
- ☐ Pre-qualify with a lender
- ☐ Interview commercial real estate broker
- ☐ Identify location
- ☐ Perform demographic study
- ☐ Interview equipment specialist
- ☐ Interview Attorney
- ☐ Interview CPA
- ☐ Interview startup consultants

B. Location Identified

- ☐ Submit letter of intent (LOI)
- ☐ Perform site analysis with help of equipment specialist
- ☐ Ensure that 200 amps of power exist
- ☐ Ensure that location is zoned for medical/dental

C. Landlord Accepts Your LOI

- ☐ Interview architects
- ☐ Submit credentialing paperwork to insurance companies
- ☐ Submit paperwork for life insurance, disability, malpractice and general liability, among others, to insurance broker
- ☐ Attorney negotiates lease
- ☐ Establish legal structure
- ☐ Select equipment specialist

D. Lease is signed

- ☐ Architect is selected & attorney reviews architect contract

- [ ] Finalized blueprints are submitted to Contractors for bids, and attorney reviews contractor contract

E. One Month Before Office Opening

- [ ] Setup QuickBooks file and bookkeeping structure with CPA
- [ ] Contact HR for Health for new hire employee documents and employee handbook.
- [ ] Submit fictitious business name application
- [ ] Submit applications to dental board
- [ ] Submit oral conscious sedation or general anesthesia permit
- [ ] Create Marketing Plan
- [ ] Open bank account
- [ ] Apply for National Provider Identifier number
- [ ] Begin designing website
- [ ] Design business cards, logo, stationery, etc.
- [ ] Apply for National Provider Identifier number
- [ ] Begin designing website
- [ ] Design business cards, logo, stationery, etc.

About the Author

Ali Oromchian, J.D., LL.M. is one of the nation's leading dental lawyers on topics relevant to dentists.

He's the founder of the Dental and Medical Counsel P.C. law firm which is regarded as one of the preeminent dental law firms devoted to dental entrepreneurs.

His clients seek his advice on practice acquisitions and sales, creation of corporations and partnerships, associate contracts, estate planning, employment law matters, office leasing and state board defense.

He also founded HR for Health, winner of the prestigious 2016 Best of Class Award, which is the leader in providing web-based human resources solutions and advice for dentists ensuring HR compliance for dental practices, protecting them from employment law risks.

HR for Health provides solutions including automated workflows for employment documentation required for compliance, customized employee handbooks, performance management tools backed by metrics, strategic time and attendance tracking, real-time benefits tracking, recurring task management, a cloud-based document vault and access to health care focused HR specialists & HR attorneys.

 Mr. Oromchian is recognized as an exceptional speaker and educator that simplifies complex legal topics and has lectured extensively throughout the United States, including to the American Dental

Association, California Dental Association, and the American Association of Orthodontists, among other.

He is also a frequent guest lecturer at local dental societies and study groups. He is frequently quoted and has written articles for the California Dental Association, Progressive Dentist, Progressive Orthodontists, and The New Dentist magazines.

Mr. Oromchian is a member of the California and District of Columbia Bar.

49303713R00063

Made in the USA
San Bernardino, CA
19 May 2017